I Have Wha...

15 Essential Facts to Help You Navigate Your Cancer Diagnosis

A cancer diagnosis is a game changer. It turns your world upside down. It is important get on top of this disease – right from the first day – by knowing what to do and who to contact. In this important Itty Bitty Book, Jacqueline Kreple, President of Fighters 4 Life, explains what your options are from getting a second opinion to traditional and alternative therapies. It is a book filled with important information for both cancer patients and their caregivers.

Information You Will Find In this Book:

- Why it is important to get and keep your medical records with you at all times and how to do it.
- What is meant by stages of cancer and why that is important.
- Why you should never skimp on treatment, nutrition and exercise and where to go for help if you need it.

If you or someone you know has cancer pick up this important, easy-to-read easy-to-follow book today!

Excellent!

Great book with lots of good info and links.

~ Ken

Your Amazing
Itty Bitty®
Cancer Book

15 Essential Steps to Help You Navigate
Your Cancer Diagnosis

Jacqueline C. Kreple
Fighters 4 Life

Published by Itty Bitty® Publishing
A subsidiary of S & P Productions, Inc.

Printed in the United States of America

Itty Bitty® Publishing
311 Main Street, Suite E
El Segundo, CA 90245
(310) 640-8885

ISBN: 978-1-931191-84-5

This book is dedicated to Michael and Lancing Kreple whose unwavering support and love have made this and so much more possible!

To Madison Thank you for sharing your childhood heart with me.

To my Mom Joan who has always kept pushing me along and helping me with my opportunities. Who always says, "Sure I can help," and for making this book possible.

To my Daddy Hans who has faced his own cancer diagnosis. He has always been there for me, cheering me on. I am forever grateful. I love you Daddy. To Candee, thank you for all your love and support.

To my brothers Peter and Richard. I love you.

To my aunt Suzy, thanks for making this book possible and for all the help you're going to give me in the future.

To my family in Michigan, Randy, Pat, Tom and Bobbie, Sheri and Len, Ally, Tommy and Ben. Thank you for your continued support.

To Charlie Wittmack my mentor. Thank you for always picking up the phone and having an answer. To Russ Scala for helping save my husband's life. To Dr. Ulick for being THAT doctor who was willing to go the extra mile.

If you wish to know more about dealing with cancer and cancer treatments, visit me on the Itty Bitty® Publishing Blog.

www.ittybittypublishing.com

or visit

www.fighters4life.org

Table of Contents

Introduction

A Cancer Diagnosis

Cancer is the second greatest killer-disease in the world and the numbers are rising. It is indiscriminate in its victims. It kills infants, toddlers, teens and those who appear healthy from their twenties to their nineties. It takes many forms and it no longer tends to be hereditary.

In 2015 alone, 1 in 2 women and 1 in 3 men will be expected to contract cancer. The good news is that treatments are improving every day.

The important thing to know about cancer is that you must waste no time addressing it. Cancer will not go away if you ignore it. A second important thing to know about cancer is that you don't have to look sick to have cancer.

There are many different kinds of treatment from traditional to holistic. The more of them you embrace, the better your chances of surviving this dreadful disease.

The 15 Facts covered in this Amazing Itty Bitty® Book are where you start when you first receive a diagnosis of cancer. What you need to know is that Michael Kreple, my husband, was diagnosed with Non-Hodgkins Lymphoma at the age of 40 and was given 30 days to live. Today he is in full remission. That's why, as soon as you can, it's essential to get into the mindframe that thinks, "There is always hope."

Fighters 4 Life, the non-profit I founded to help other people like us battle this disease, exists to support cancer patients and their caregivers, emotionally and financially. Right now we are looking for volunteers and donors. Visit our website to learn more about us.

<u>www.fighters4life.org</u>

Simple Facts

Fact 1
Do Not Go On the Internet – Yet

The first inclination on receiving a cancer diagnosis is to turn to the internet to research your signs and symptoms and their possible outcome. Wait until you get a diagnosis from an oncology team. There are many facts and statistics available on the internet, but they are not always accurate in terms of *your* diagnosis. These facts and statistics may be very scary, but they also might not apply to you.

1. Wait to learn what stage of cancer you have.
2. Wait to learn what the protocol is. By that I mean, what does your oncology team suggest in terms of treatment?

Every patient is an individual. Every patient's cancer is individual. The way one person responds to treatment is not necessarily the way you will respond to the same treatment for the same disease. Don't assume that what is described on the internet is going to be the same experience or outcome for you.

The Time Frame

The time frame for a diagnosis depends on any number of factors, including:

- The kind of insurance you have.
- What kinds of tests are required to make a definitive diagnosis.
- Your oncology team.
- Your signs and symptoms.
- Your history.

Fact 2
You *Can* Get a Second Opinion

Many people are inclined to stay with the oncology team that diagnosed them. There is a certain degree of comfort and trust in that relationship. However, if you have any questions or concerns regarding your oncology team and their protocol, it's okay to get a second opinion.

1. Getting a second opinion is your right as a cancer patient if:
    a. You have doubts about your doctor.
    b. You don't get along with your doctor.
    c. Your doctor doesn't have much experience treating your kind of cancer.
    d. You have a rare cancer and need a specialty team.
    e. Your doctor says there is no lifesaving therapy available.
2. Seeking a second opinion is an option, not a requirement.
3. Seeking a second opinion is actually increasingly common.
4. The second opinion can confirm the direction in which you are already heading, and it might also suggest new directions or considerations.
5. It's important to be proactive in your cancer care.

How to Get A Second Opinion.

- Start by asking your primary care physician for another recommendation.
- If your doctor seems bothered by your asking for a second opinion, you should definitely get one. Good doctors want you to feel confident in their care.
- Getting a second opinion does not mean giving up your original oncology team – it means getting a second opinion.
- If you ask for a second opinion, your doctor should say, "Good idea. Here's a list of names."
- In some cases, a third opinion might be helpful, particularly if your specialists can't agree on a course of treatment.
    - For example, if you have prostate cancer and your oncologist and urologist do not agree.

Fact 3
Let Your Family Know and Get
All the Support You Need

It's important to have a good support team in your corner; you'll need that. Whether it be family, friends or support groups within your cancer community – it takes a village.

1. There are no wrong ways to tell your family what's going on. You can tell them right away or wait until you have all the information (i.e. diagnosis and protocol).
2. You should never feel like a burden. Support is there to help you navigate and facilitate your cancer journey.
3. Supporters are honored by your request for help.
4. Sometimes, even with a great deal of support, the cancer battle is very lonely.

Support groups include:

- Your caregiver
- Your family and friends
- The community in which you live and thrive
- Your cancer community
- Non-profits aimed at helping cancer patients

Fact 4
Remember That the Doctor
Has To Focus On the Disease

When you get your protocol from your oncology team, their goal is to treat the cancer. Many protocols or treatments leave the patient really sick. Be sure to keep your primary care physician informed and up to date – especially if you are finding yourself in and out of the ER.

1. Many of the suggested nutrition concepts, in my opinion, are outrageous. What the medical community wants to do is treat symptoms and side effects with more medication, rather than with nutrition and exercise.
2. Oncologists focus on the cancer, they have a team to focus on the patient.
3. They don't deal with the self-image problems caused by the loss of hair resulting from cancer treatment.
4. Many treatment protocols have adverse long term effects, such as heart damage. That means that you are sent from one specialist to another. All your doctors should meet regularly to discuss your progress and treatment.

How to Maintain a Healthy Patient

There are many questions in this current medical modality regarding the care and treatment of cancer patients.

- During cancer treatment, you need to stay hydrated. Many treatment protocols are hard on other organs like your kidneys and it is important to keep your system flushed.
- During cancer treatment, you need to eat well and maintain a healthy weight.
- You might need help coping with the emotional impact of cancer.
- While your doctor's main focus is on the cancer, there are other health professionals who will work hard to keep the rest of you healthy.
- Utilize your caregiver, family, oncology nurse, case, patient navigator or social worker and cancer community to help you navigate health.
- Your oncology nurses often spend far more time with you than your doctor does, answering questions and caring for you.
- Your social worker can also help you find resources from alternative doctors to non-profits.
- For many people, faith, prayer and meditation are important for getting through treatment. Advisors in this area include priests, ministers, rabbis or spiritual advisors.

Fact 5
Stages of Cancer

"The term 'Stage of Cancer' means the point the cancer was at when it was first diagnosed. Being sure about the stage is critical, because it determines the best way to decide your treatment plan. On average, the higher the stage, the worse the effect of the cancer on the person who has it."

~ Cancer Institute NSW

1. Stage 0 – *In situ*. Cancer in the position where it started. Most likely this kind of cancer never goes beyond this stage.
2. Stage 1 – Localized Spread. The cancer cells gain the ability to spread to the neighboring tissue.
3. Stages 2 & 3 – Regional Spread. The cancer has spread to the general region in which it began, but not to other parts of the body.
4. Stage 4 – Distant Spread. Once it goes into the blood stream, it can travel almost anywhere in the body and form new colonies.

~Cancer Treatment Centers Of America

Information About the Stages of Cancer

If you want to read more about the stages of cancer, here are some worthwhile sites to visit.

- The American Cancer Society
- Saint Jude Children's Hospital
- About.com
- Cancer Centers of America
- The society for your specific type of cancer; for example, The Leukemia and Lymphoma Society.

Fact 6
The Grades of Cancer

The term "Grades of Cancer" describes the look of the cells.

1. Grade 1. Cancer cells that resemble normal cells and are not growing rapidly.
2. Grade 2. Cancer cells that don't look like normal cells and are growing faster than normal cells.
3. Grade 3. Cancer cells that look abnormal and may grow or spread aggressively.

~Cancer Center of America

The Grades of Cancer

To learn more about grades of cancer, visit:

- The American Cancer Society
- Saint Jude's Children's Hospital
- About.com
- Cancer Centers of America
- The society for your specific type of cancer; for example, in our case it was The Leukemia and Lymphoma Society

Fact 7
Making a Treatment Decision

Making a treatment decision involves many steps, all of which are part of navigating your cancer treatment.

Treatment decisions include:

1. Understanding your diagnosis.
2. Knowing your treatment options.
3. Understanding the goals of your treatment.
4. Knowing the side effects of each treatment option.
5. Considering the risks and benefits of each treatment option.
6. Finding help managing the cost of your cancer care.
7. Finding help managing the costs of everyday living for yourself and your family while you are undergoing treatment.
8. Discussing your decisions with people you trust.

Making a Treatment Decision

If you are unfamiliar with some of the words being used by your oncology team, this is a good time to access on-line information.

- If you go to the American Cancer Society and type in the word you don't understand, you will be given a good definition or explanation.
- Ask your oncology nurse or social worker.
- Cancercenter.com (The Cancer Centers of America) has a lot of good information for you.

Make sure you understand everything that's being said to you.

Fact 8
Traditional Treatments

Traditional treatment means those treatments performed by medical doctors and specialists in oncology. The following explains some of them:

1. Chemotherapy is an important part of treatment for many patients. You may receive chemotherapy alone or in combination with other modalities.
2. Radiation Therapy is also an important part of treatment for some patients. Its object is to shrink the tumor, while limiting the treatments impact on surrounding cells.
3. Surgical Oncology depends on factors such as type, size, location, grade and stage of tumor. For many patients, surgical oncology will be combined with other cancer treatments. Not all patients have operable cancers.
4. Hormone Therapy is a form of systemic (the whole body) treatment which works to add, block or remove hormones from the body to slow or remove cancer cells.

How to Manage Some Effects of Traditional Treatments

A word about managing the side effects of Chemotherapy.

- While Chemotherapy targets cancer cells, it can also damage other rapidly growing cells, like the lining of your stomach and cause unpleasant side effects.
- These unpleasant effects include, but are not limited to: nausea, vomiting, hair loss, fatigue, chemo brain (an inability to stay focused) and mouth sores.
- Make sure that you stay hydrated and keep your electrolytes up.
- You can take anti-nausea medication.
- Herbal teas can help soothe your stomach and keep you hydrated.
- It's important to maintain healthy nutrition, but if you are vomiting most foods and you find a food you can keep down, eat that.
- Three to five days after every treatment, take a very hot bath containing 1 cup of aluminum free baking soda and 1 cup of sea salt. This process will pull toxins and chemicals from your body.

Fact 9
Treatments Beyond Chemo and Radiation

There are many kinds of traditional medical treatments beyond chemotherapy, radiation and surgery that you may not have heard of. Some of these include:

1. Immunotherapy, also called Biological Therapy and Bio Therapy, uses your immune system to fight cancer. It either stimulates your immune system to attack cancer cells or provides your immune system with antibodies to fight specific kinds of cancer.
2. Hematologic Oncology addresses blood cancers. It is a specialized therapy that uses a powerful combination of treatments, such as aggressive chemotherapy and advanced radiation. It also uses stem cell transplantation to help the blood replace cancerous blood cells with healthy blood cells.
3. Neurosurgery is a specialized practice for cancers of the nervous system and its supporting structures (spine). A neurological team includes a neurosurgeon, radiation oncologist, medical oncologist, pathologist, psychologist, rehabilitation therapist and possibly other experts.

Cancer is a General Term for Many Different Forms of This Disease

Cancer is a general term for many different forms of this disease. Your cancer diagnosis will determine what kind of doctors your team will be comprised of.

- It is important that you understand that you have assembled the correct team.
  - What kind of cancer do I have?
  - Has the correct team been assembled?
  - What is the specific role that each member of my team plays?
  - Have I asked the right questions about all my options?
- For example, it is a good thing to get a specialist in Hematologic Oncology if you have a blood cancer.

Fact 10
Cancer Drugs to Clinical Trials

More traditional treatments for different forms of cancer include:

1. Cancer Drugs – or chemotherapy drugs often used in combinations of 2, 3 or 4. For example, the chemotherapy drug combinations – "The Chop," includes cyclophosphamide, doxorubicin, vincristine and prednisone. There are many other combinations of cancer drugs.
2. Interventional Radiology is a minimally invasive treatment. This is generally used in: colorectal, breast, gall bladder, pancreas, lung, and esophageal cancers, as well as stomach melanomas and sarcomas, to name just a few.
3. Clinical Trials – many hospitals are committed to bringing new and innovative investigational cancer treatment options to the market. Research or ask your oncologist which particular hospitals and cancer centers are involved in these kinds of trials. Clinical Trials are usually sought out when there are no standard treatments available for your type of cancer.

~Cancer Treatment Centers of America

Information on Clinical Trials

Information about Clinical Trials is available online.

- Cancer Treatment Centers of America can provide a list of clinical trials across America.
- You can email Clinicaltrials@ctca-hope.com and ask what clinical trials are available for which type of cancer.
- Tigertrials.com/nsclc
- www.cancer.gov/aboutcancer/treatment/clinical-trials
- www.cancer.org/ssLINK/clinical-trials-landing.

For more information, Google "clinical trials" for a complete list.

Fact 11
Doing Your Holistic Research

Naturopathic medicine is a great supplement to Allopathic (traditional) Medicine. Naturopathic medicine includes, but is not limited to:

1. AutoHemo Therapy, which boosts your immune system, decreases inflammation and increases oxygenation at the tissue level. Blood is taken from your arm, exposed to ozone gas, then returned to the body.
2. Heavy Metal detoxification uses various natural methods to bind these toxins so they can be eliminated safely from the body.
3. High Doses of Vitamin C Therapy. Vitamin C is one of the safest and most effective nutrients. It is a powerful antioxidant. Its benefits include immune enhancement, protection from viruses and bacteria, cardiovascular protection, eye disease and healthy skin. When taken in high doses (IV Vitamin C), it has been known to kill cancer cells. When taken orally in recommended doses, it acts as an antioxidant, destroying free radicals. Note: Vitamin C supplements can reduce the effectiveness of many cancer drugs.

~ WebMD.com

Vitamin C, Oxygen, Alkalinity and More

Some vitamins, minerals and herbs help the body fight cancer. Some may interfere with treatment and should be managed accordingly.

- Vitamin C should NEVER be taken on the day of traditional cancer treatment or for five days following that treatment.
- Cesium, Rubimius and Potassium, in this combination, are able to enter cancer cells, changing their Ph from acid to alkaline.
- Cancer does not do well in a well-oxygenated body.
- Cancer does not do well in a body with a high alkaline Ph.
- Cancer thrives on sugar, so keep your sugar intake low. Processed foods like bread, white rice, canned or packaged foods turn rapidly into sugar, so avoid them.
- Cancer loves stress, so try to find ways to reduce those stress levels (meditation, prayer, hypnosis and so forth).

Fact 12
Doing More Holistic Research

1. Lymphatic Massage. The Lymphatic system is often called the body's garbage collector. It collects and eliminates waste from the body every morning and is a crucial part of the body's immune system – which is why exercise in the morning is so beneficial. Lymphatic Massage helps remove wastes and toxins from your body through the lymph fluid.
2. Juicing raw vegetables and fruits provides enzymes, vitamins, antioxidants and phytochemicals, which can offer benefits in so many ways. Each phytochemical works differently.
3. Exercise is a different experience for all cancer patients. It can be a challenge, according to how you are reacting to your treatment protocol. Any exercise is beneficial and should be taken into consideration, no matter how difficult it may be.
4. Survivorship Support and group therapies are really important in the healing process. They help you move forward without guilt, both for the cancer survivor and the caregivers of survivors, or if you have lost a loved one.

~Utopia Wellness

Where to Do Your Holistic Research

These are just a few of the many places that are available. Contact them, ask questions and find the right alternative cancer treatment provider for your own needs.

This list covers just a few of the holistic options; there are many, many more.

- The Institute of Nutritional Medicine and Cardiovascular Research. Directed by Russ Scalla. You can look him up on YouTube under Russ Scalla.
  www.personalizedhealthinstitute.com
- This website is easy to use and the information is excellent.
  www.utopiawellness.com.

Fact 13
Record Keeping

In many cases, when you are in the doctor's office the information can be so overwhelming that you are physically unable to digest or even hear what the doctor is saying. Many people leave these visits more confused than they were when they went in.

1. Have your caregiver and/or a recording device with you at all visits. Generally speaking, doctors will not like you recording your visit, so use discretion.

Create your portable filing system.

1. Following every visit, print out or request a printout of your medical records.
2. Keep them in a portable filing system which you should carry with you to every doctor's visit, as well as whenever you are traveling.
3. Many people think that with current technology doctors have easy-access to medical records. This is not so; it can take days for a new team of doctors to receive current medical information.
4. This record includes every scan, blood draw, biopsy, MRI and doctor's visit.

Record Keeping

Although your records are in digital format, medical records departments are constantly getting medical records requests and you are put into the order in which your requests are received.

To Create a Record System Use:

- A portable accordion file with a handle is the best choice.
- Get the numbered rather than the alphabetical file.
- Organize it by date. You can separate out different years by putting them in different, dated, manila files.

Fact 14
Financial Burden

Managing the cost of treatment is difficult for many patients and families coping with cancer. Finances can make it more difficult to follow a doctor's treatment plan.

1. Many times the reality of cost doesn't sink in until you are undergoing treatment.
2. Finances can leave you thinking less about recovery and more about how you're going to pay for treatment.
3. Many people dealing with financial concerns, especially out of pocket payment costs, tend to drop their treatment in the middle of it.
4. Almost 46% of patients dealing with the financial burden of cancer care cut back on necessary expenses such as food to pay for cancer treatment.

Do not skimp on your treatment or on healthy food – there is help.

Financial Assistance

Here are some ways to find financial assistance.

- Your social worker/caseworker has many resources where you can find financial assistance.
- The American Cancer Society Health Insurance Assistance Service. (800) ACS-2345
- CancerCare Co-Payment Assistance Foundation. They cover the cost of co-payments to help with the cost of medication for certain cancers.
- HealthWell Foundation – which helps patients cover their out-of-pocket medical expenses.

Drug Assistance Programs

- NeedyMeds.
- The Partnership For Prescription Assistance.
- Pharmaceutical companies have programs featuring their patented drugs and can offer access and discounts. Contact the provider directly.
- Provider Discount Charity Care. Some doctors and hospitals may be willing to give patients a break, but the patients must ask.

Fact 15
Reach Out to Your Cancer Society and Non-Profits For Help

Now you can go on the Internet. Now you can start researching based on your diagnosis, staging and treatment protocol, but be aware that some of the information can be overwhelming and scary and not necessarily applicable to you and your journey.

Contact:
1. The American Cancer Society.
2. Cancer Cares.
3. The organizations that address your particular cancer.
4. There are many, many non-profit cancer related organizations out there to help you, but you have to really search for them.
5. Reach out to www.fighters4life.org, as they offer both emotional and financial support.

Remember in Cancer More Than The Patient May Need Help.

When a member of a family gets cancer the whole family gets cancer. It is important to make certain that everyone has their needs met.

- Children often blame themselves when a parent gets cancer. It's normal but shouldn't be ignored.
- If one child gets cancer the other children may suffer from feelings of abandonment as attention shifts intensely to their sibling.
- If a parent gets cancer children sometimes feel as if they are being robbed of the attention that should be theirs.
- Parents blame themselves when their children get cancer.
- The strain on caregivers is immense as they tend to forget themselves and their own needs as they focus all their attention on their patient.

It is very important to make sure that everyone's psychological needs are met. Make sure you reach out to friends, relatives, your community and organizations within your community. Reach out to Fighters4Life. Support is what we do.

The Kinds of Things Fighters 4 Life Has Helped With

To name a few of the things that Jacky Kreple and Fighters 4 Life do:

- We have helped Cancer Fighters from age 2 to age 80, each according to what they need.
- We support Cancer Fighters with financial aid during treatment.
- Jacky Kreple spent a week in a hotel in Chicago with a woman who was receiving radiation of her eye. She didn't want her to be alone.
- She has spent nights and days in emergency rooms supporting cancer patients.
- She goes to doctor's appointments with cancer patients, whether the appointments are surgery, checkups or chemotherapy.
- Jacky is a cancer coach. She coaches cancer patients, caregivers and their families through their cancer journeys – whether it's to remission or the passing of a loved one.
- Fighters 4 Life has teamed up with other organizations to help bring the first Cancer Treatment Center to the horn of Africa in Tanzania.
- We are currently researching the possibility of bringing preventative treatment and awareness of cervical cancer to Indonesia.

You've finished. Before you go…

<u>Tweet/share that you finished this book.</u>
Please star rate this book.
Reviews are solid gold to writers. Please
take a few minutes to give us some itty bitty
feedback.

ABOUT THE AUTHOR

Jacqueline and Michael Kreple, an athletic, physically fit, young couple with young children, never considered facing a life-changing event like cancer.

To their shock and dismay Michael, a Mixed Martial Arts fighter preparing for his second fight, was diagnosed with Non-Hodgkins Lymphoma and given 30 days to live. In that moment he stepped into the cancer ring to begin the fight of his life. Without insurance, the first emergency room visit cost them $44,000.

Michael and Jacqueline qualified for MediCal, but it was a weekly fight to keep it. Without that insurance, Michael would have died within the first month of his diagnosis.

The next two years were the battle of a lifetime as Jacky fought to keep her husband on MediCal and Michael fought to stay alive. She researched every possible kind of therapy available to them. They embraced traditional and holistic therapies alike, refusing to leave one possibility untried. Jacky changed the family diet completely, learned how to give injections – even grew flats of wheat grass, while Michael tried to maintain his fitness between treatments.

Their friends rallied around them, throwing one fundraiser after another to help them meet the expenses of daily life when Michael was undergoing treatment. These friends said they very much enjoyed fundraising because they could see where their efforts were going.

It was during this time that Jacky decided to dedicate herself to helping other cancer patients when this ordeal was over. Her dream was to create relationships between donors and the cancer patients they help so they can see and share in the experience of the help they provide.

Today, Michael is cancer-free and Jacky has created Fighters 4 Life, a non-profit organization dedicated to supporting cancer patients, their families and caregivers – emotionally and physically. It raises funds to help them meet the on-going expenses of everyday life during treatment and is creating classes to teach others how to support cancer patients and their caregivers.

www.fighters4life.org

**If You Liked This Book
You Might Also Enjoy….**

- **Your Amazing Itty Bitty® Gratitude Book** – Belinda Lee Cook

- **Your Amazing Itty Bitty® Marijuana Manual** – Kat Bohnsack

- **Your Amazing Itty Bitty® Heal Your Body Book** – Patricia Garza Pinto

…And Many More Itty Bitty® Books in Paperback And Online.